I0703081

UNLOCKING WELLNESS

Chair Yoga for Beginners; Embracing Chair Yoga for Health and Well-being

Sarah Scott

Copyright

Copyright © 2024 by Hala Rashida

All rights reserved. No part of this publication may be reproduced, distributed, or transmitted in any form or by any means, including photocopying, recording, or other electronic or mechanical methods, without the prior written permission of the publisher, except in the case of brief quotations embodied in critical reviews and certain other noncommercial uses permitted by copyright law.

Disclaimer

The information in this book, UNLOCKING WELLNESS: Chair Yoga for Beginners; Embracing Chair Yoga for Health and Well-being, by Sarah Scott, is for informational purposes only and is not medical advice. Consult a healthcare professional before starting any new exercise program, especially if you have health concerns. The author and publisher are not responsible for any injury or harm resulting from the use of this book. Your participation is at your own risk.

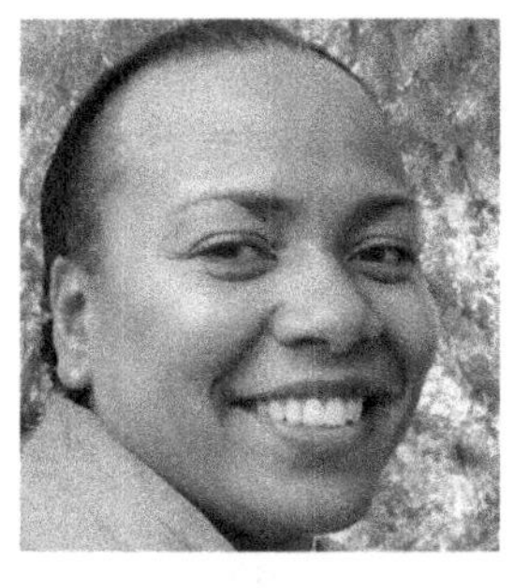 ## About the Author

Sarah Scott is a dedicated yoga instructor and wellness advocate, committed to making yoga accessible to all. With extensive experience in teaching, she specializes in chair yoga, offering a gentle and adaptable approach for individuals of all abilities. Her passion for health and well-being shines through her writing and teaching.Sarah's work aims to inspire and support people on their journey to better health. When she's not teaching or writing, she enjoys outdoor activities, mindfulness practices, and spending time with her family.

Chair yoga for beginners 6

TABLE OF CONTENTS

INTRODUCTION TO CHAIR YOGA

Chair yoga is a gentle form of yoga that is practiced sitting on a chair or using a chair for support. It offers all the benefits of traditional yoga, including improved flexibility, strength, balance, and relaxation, but in a modified format that makes it accessible to a wider range of individuals, including those with mobility issues, seniors, office workers, and people with limited flexibility.

What is Chair Yoga?

Chair yoga adapts traditional yoga poses and techniques so they can be done while seated on a chair or using a chair for support. It incorporates gentle stretches, mindful breathing exercises, and relaxation techniques to help participants experience the benefits of yoga without having to get down on the floor.

While some chair yoga classes may involve standing and using the chair for support, many poses can be done entirely while seated. Poses are modified to accommodate different levels of flexibility and mobility, making chair yoga suitable for people of all ages and fitness levels.

Benefits of Chair Yoga

1. *Improved Flexibility*: Chair yoga helps improve flexibility by gently stretching the muscles and joints, reducing stiffness and increasing range of motion.

2. *Increased Strength:* Even though chair yoga is done while seated, it still provides opportunities to strengthen muscles, particularly in the core and lower body, through isometric contractions and resistance exercises.

3. *Better Posture:* Chair yoga encourages proper alignment and awareness of posture, helping to alleviate strain on the spine and promote good posture habits.

4. *Enhanced Balance*: Practicing balance poses while seated on a chair can improve stability and proprioception, reducing the risk of falls.

5. *Stress Reduction*: Chair yoga incorporates relaxation techniques such as deep breathing and mindfulness, which can help reduce stress, anxiety, and tension

6. *Improved Circulation*: Gentle movements and stretches in chair yoga can help improve circulation, which can benefit overall health and vitality.

7. *Accessible Exercise*: Chair yoga is accessible to people of all ages and fitness levels, including those with mobility issues, chronic pain, or physical limitations. It can be done at home, in the office, or in a group setting, making it a convenient option for many.

8. *Mind-Body Connection*: Like traditional yoga, chair yoga emphasizes the connection between the mind and body, promoting a sense of inner calm, self-awareness, and overall well-being.

Who Can Benefit from Chair Yoga?

Seniors: Chair yoga is particularly beneficial for seniors who may have limited mobility or difficulty getting up and down from the floor. It provides a safe and gentle way to stay active, maintain flexibility, and promote overall health and well-being.

Office Workers: People who spend long hours sitting at a desk can benefit from incorporating chair yoga into their daily routine to counteract the effects of prolonged sitting, reduce muscle tension, and improve posture and circulation.

Individuals with Mobility Issues: Chair yoga offers a safe and accessible form of exercise for individuals with mobility issues, chronic pain, arthritis, or other physical limitations. Poses can be modified to accommodate specific needs and abilities.

Beginners: Chair yoga is a great introduction to yoga for beginners or those who are new to exercise. It provides a gentle and supportive environment to learn basic yoga poses, breathing techniques, and mindfulness practices.

Anyone Looking for a Gentle Exercise Option: Whether recovering from injury, managing a chronic condition, or simply looking for a low-impact exercise option, chair yoga offers a gentle yet effective way to improve physical fitness, reduce stress, and promote overall health and well-being.

In summary, chair yoga is a versatile and accessible form of exercise that offers numerous physical, mental, and emotional benefits. By making yoga more inclusive and adaptable, chair yoga empowers individuals of all ages and abilities to experience the transformative power of yoga in their daily lives

GETTING STARTED WITH CHAIR YOGA

Getting started with chair yoga is easy and requires minimal equipment or experience. In this chapter, we'll cover everything you need to know to begin your chair yoga practice, including finding the right chair, preparing your space, and understanding basic chair yoga etiquette.

Finding the Right Clothes

When practicing chair yoga, wearing the right clothes ensures comfort and ease of movement. Here are some tips:

1. Comfortable and Breathable: Choose clothing made of breathable fabrics like cotton or moisture-wicking materials to stay cool and dry during practice.

2. *Stretchy and Flexible:* Opt for stretchy materials such as spandex or elastane that allow for unrestricted movement, especially important for seated poses in chair yoga.

3. *Fitted but Not Restrictive:* Wear fitted clothing that moves with your body but doesn't constrict your movements, ensuring comfort and ease during practice.

4. *Avoid Tight Waistbands:* Avoid wearing anything tight around the waist to prevent discomfort or restriction of movement, allowing you to fully engage in chair yoga poses.

5. *Simple Design*: Choose simple designs without excessive zippers, buttons, or embellishments to minimize distractions and ensure focus on the practice.

Finding the Right Chair

When practicing chair yoga, it's important to choose a chair that is sturdy, stable, and comfortable. Here are some tips for finding the right chair:

1. *Sturdy Construction:* Choose a chair with a solid frame and stable legs to ensure safety and support during your practice.

2. *Comfortable Seat:* Look for a chair with a padded seat cushion that provides comfort and allows you to sit for an extended period without discomfort.

3. *Appropriate Height:* The height of the chair should allow your feet to rest flat on the floor with your knees bent at a 90-degree angle. Avoid chairs that are too high or too low, as they can cause strain on your joints.

4. Armrests: While not necessary, chairs with armrests can provide additional support and stability during certain poses.

5. Adjustable Features: If possible, choose a chair with adjustable features such as height or armrests, allowing you to customize it to your specific needs and preferences.

6. Non-Slip Surface: Ensure that the chair's feet have non-slip grips to prevent sliding or slipping during your practice.

Preparing Your Space

Setting up a dedicated space for your chair yoga practice can help create a peaceful and conducive environment for relaxation and focus. Here's how to prepare your space:

1. *Clearing the Area:* Choose a quiet, clutter-free area with enough room to move comfortably around your chair. Remove any obstacles or distractions that may interfere with your practice.

2. *Comfortable Atmosphere*: Set the mood for your practice by dimming the lights, playing soft music, or lighting candles or incense to create a calming ambiance.

3. *Props and Accessories:* Gather any props or accessories you may need for your practice, such as yoga blocks, straps, or pillows, and have them nearby for easy access.

4. *Personalize Your Space:* Add personal touches to your practice space, such as photos, inspirational quotes, or decorative items that bring you joy and help you feel relaxed and centered.

5. Safety Considerations: Ensure that your practice space is safe and free from hazards such as loose rugs or cords. If practicing near furniture or walls, be mindful of your surroundings to avoid accidental bumps or collisions.

Basic Chair Yoga Etiquette

Just like any other yoga class, chair yoga has its own set of etiquette guidelines to ensure a positive and respectful experience for everyone. Here are some basic chair yoga etiquette tips to keep in mind:

1. Arrive on Time: Arrive a few minutes early to set up your space and settle in before the class begins. If you need to leave early, inform the instructor beforehand and try to do so discreetly to minimize disruption.

2. Respect Personal Space: Be mindful of the personal space of others in the class and avoid encroaching on their area. Keep your belongings neatly organized and avoid placing them in a way that obstructs others' movement.

3. Listen to Your Body: Honor your body's limits and avoid pushing yourself into discomfort or pain. If a pose doesn't feel right for you, feel free to modify or skip it altogether. Focus on your own practice without comparing yourself to others.

4. Keep Noise to a Minimum: Respect the peaceful atmosphere of the class by keeping conversation and distractions to a minimum. Silence your phone and refrain from talking during the practice to maintain a tranquil environment.

5. *Follow the Instructor's Guidance:* Pay attention to the instructor's cues and follow their guidance throughout the class. If you have any questions or concerns, don't hesitate to ask for clarification or assistance.

By finding the right chair, preparing your space, and adhering to basic chair yoga etiquette, you can set yourself up for a successful and enjoyable chair yoga practice. With these foundational elements in place, you're ready to embark on your journey toward improved health, relaxation, and well-being through chair yoga.

CHAIR YOGA WARM-UP SEQUENCE

A chair yoga warm-up sequence is designed to gently prepare the body for movement, increase blood flow, and improve flexibility. Here's an extensive chair yoga warm-up sequence:

1. Seated Breathing (2-3 minutes): Sit tall on the chair, close your eyes, and focus on your breath. Inhale deeply through the nose, filling your lungs, and exhale completely through the mouth. Repeat for several breaths.

2. Neck Stretches (1 minute): Drop your right ear towards your right shoulder, feeling a stretch along the left side of your neck. Hold for a few breaths, then switch sides. Repeat 2-3 times on each side.

3. Shoulder Rolls (1 minute): Roll your shoulders up, back, and down in a smooth circular motion. Reverse the direction after a few repetitions. This helps release tension in the shoulders and upper back.

4. Seated Cat-Cow Stretch (1 minute): Place your hands on your knees. Inhale, arch your back, and lift your chest (Cow Pose). Exhale, round your spine, and tuck your chin to your chest (Cat Pose). Repeat for several breaths, moving with your breath.

5. Gentle Side Bends (1 minute): Inhale, reach your right arm overhead, and exhale, gently lean to the left, stretching the right side of your body. Inhale back to center and switch sides. Repeat 2-3 times on each side.

6. Seated Forward Fold (1 minute): Inhale, lengthen your spine, and exhale, hinge forward at your hips, folding your torso over your thighs. Hold onto your shins or ankles for support. Relax your neck and shoulders. Hold for a few breaths.

7. Wrist and Ankle Circles (1 minute): Extend your arms in front of you and circle your wrists in one direction, then the other. Repeat with your ankles. This helps improve mobility in the wrists and ankles, important for many yoga poses.

8. Seated Twist (1 minute): Sit tall, inhale, and lengthen your spine. Exhale, twist to the right, placing your left hand on the outside of your right thigh and your right hand on the back of the chair. Hold for a few breaths, then switch sides.

CHAIR YOGA POSES

Chair yoga poses are modified versions of traditional yoga poses that can be performed while sitting on a chair or using a chair for support. In this chapter, we'll explore a variety of chair yoga poses that target different areas of the body and promote flexibility, strength, and relaxation.

Seated Mountain Pose

Description: Seated Mountain Pose, also known as Tadasana, is a foundational yoga pose that promotes alignment, grounding, and awareness of posture.

How to Perform:

1. Sit tall on the edge of your chair with your feet hip-width apart and flat on the floor.

2. Lengthen your spine, lift your chest, and relax your shoulders down away from your ears.

3. Place your hands on your thighs or let them rest lightly on your knees.

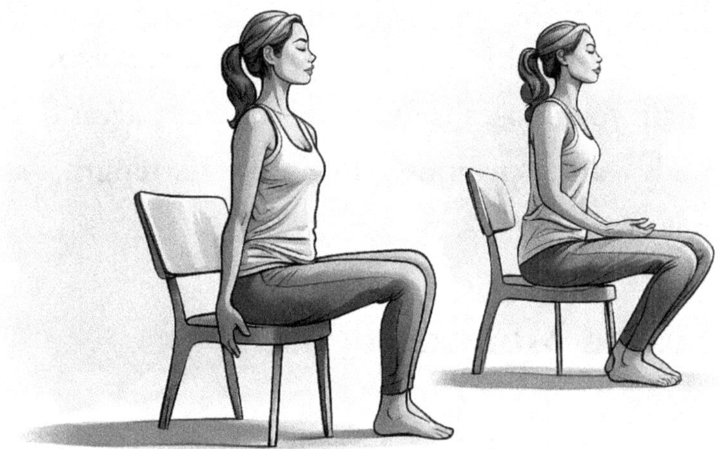

4. Close your eyes if comfortable, and take slow, deep breaths, focusing on rooting down through your sit bones and lengthening up through the crown of your head.

Benefits:

- Improves posture and alignment.
- Increases awareness of breath and body.
- Promotes a sense of grounding and stability.

Seated Forward Bend

Description: Seated Forward Bend, or Paschimottanasana, stretches the hamstrings, lower back, and spine, promoting relaxation and releasing tension.

How to Perform:
1. Sit tall on the edge of your chair with your feet flat on the floor and legs together.
2. Inhale and lengthen your spine, then exhale and hinge forward at your hips, leading with your

chest.

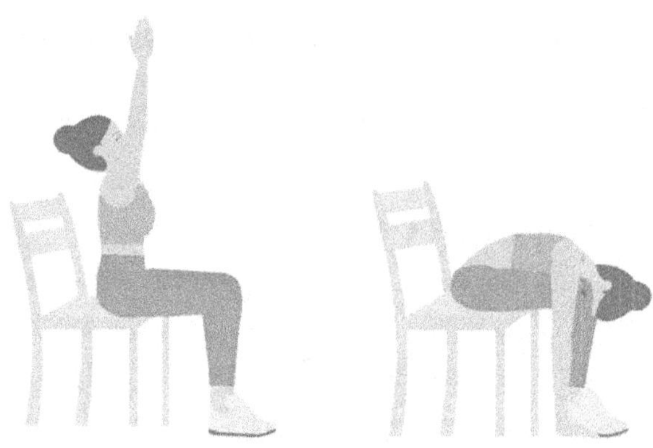

3. Allow your hands to rest on your thighs, shins, or ankles, depending on your flexibility.

4. Keep your spine long and avoid rounding your back excessively.

5. Hold the pose for several breaths, then slowly release and return to an upright position.

***Benefits*:**

- Stretches the spine, hamstrings, and lower back.

- Relieves tension and stress in the back and shoulders.
- Calms the mind and promotes relaxation.

Seated Twist

Description: Seated Twist, or Ardha Matsyendrasana, increases spinal mobility and stimulates digestion while releasing tension in the back and shoulders.

How to Perform:
1. Sit tall on the edge of your chair with your feet flat on the floor and knees together.
2. Inhale and lengthen your spine, then exhale and twist to the right, placing your left hand on the outside of your right thigh and your right

hand on the back of the chair.

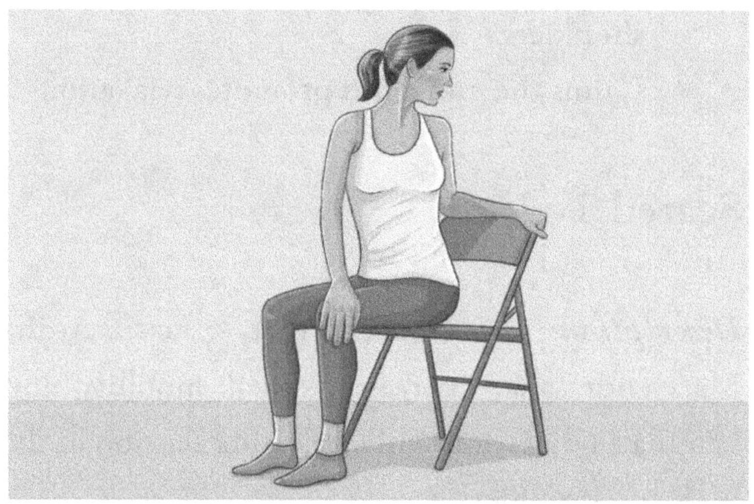

3. Keep both sit bones grounded and lengthen through your spine as you twist.

4. Hold the twist for several breaths, then inhale to release and return to center.

5. Repeat on the other side, twisting to the left.

Benefits:

- Increases spinal mobility and flexibility.
- Stimulates digestion and massages internal organs.

- Releases tension in the back, shoulders, and neck.

Seated Cat-Cow Stretch

Description: Seated Cat-Cow Stretch combines two classic yoga poses to promote spinal mobility, flexibility, and relaxation.

How to Perform:

1. Sit tall on the edge of your chair with your feet flat on the floor and hands resting on your thighs.

2. Inhale and arch your back, lifting your chest and tilting your pelvis forward (Cow Pose).

3. Exhale and round your spine, tucking your chin to your chest and drawing your belly button

toward your spine (Cat Pose).

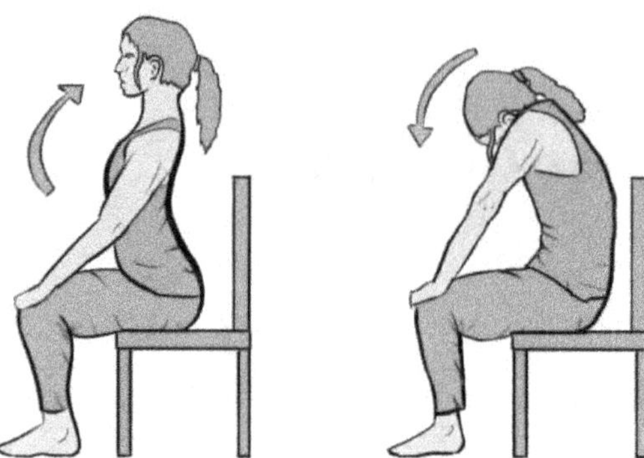

4. Continue flowing between Cat and Cow Poses with your breath, moving slowly and mindfully.

Benefits:

- Increases spinal flexibility and mobility.
- Relieves tension in the back, shoulders, and neck.
- Promotes relaxation and awareness of breath and body.

Seated Warrior Pose

Description: Seated Warrior Pose, or Virabhadrasana, strengthens the legs, core, and arms while promoting stability and focus.

How to Perform:
1. Sit tall on the edge of your chair with your feet hip-width apart and flat on the floor.
2. Extend your right leg out to the side, keeping your foot flat on the floor and toes pointing forward.
3. Bend your left knee and shift your weight slightly toward your left foot, engaging your core for stability.

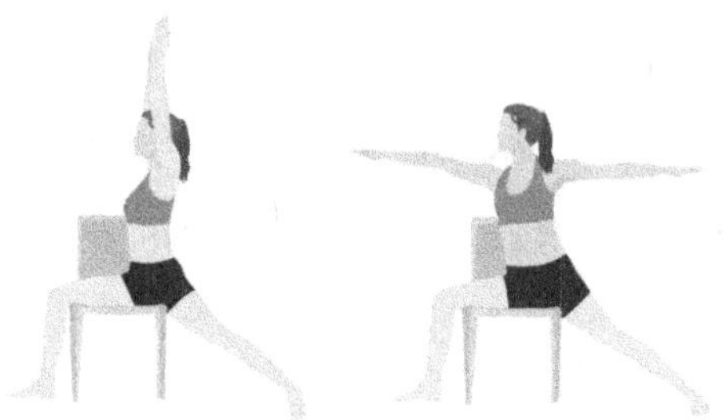

4. Extend your arms overhead, reaching toward the ceiling with your fingertips.

5. Hold the pose for several breaths, then return to center and repeat on the other side.

***Benefits*:**

- Strengthens the legs, core, and arms.
- Improves balance, stability, and focus.
- Energizes the body and promotes a sense of empowerment.

Seated Sun Salutation

Description: Seated Sun Salutation is a modified version of the traditional Sun Salutation sequence that warms up the body, increases circulation, and promotes flexibility and mindfulness.

How to Perform:
1. Sit tall on the edge of your chair with your feet flat on the floor and hands resting on your thighs.
2. Inhale and sweep your arms overhead, reaching up toward the ceiling (Mountain Pose).
3. Exhale and fold forward at your hips, bringing your hands down toward your feet (Forward Fold).
4. Inhale and lift halfway up, lengthening your spine and reaching your chest forward (Half Forward Fold).

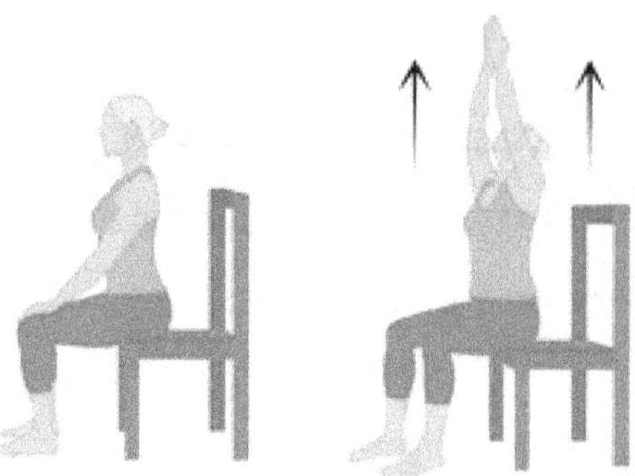

5. Exhale and fold forward again, bringing your hands back to the floor (Forward Fold).

6. Inhale and sweep your arms out to the sides and up overhead, coming back to Mountain Pose.

7. Exhale and bring your hands down to your heart center, closing your eyes and taking a moment to center and ground yourself.

***Benefits*:**

- Warms up the body and increases circulation.

- Promotes flexibility and mobility in the spine, shoulders, and hamstrings.
- Cultivates mindfulness and awareness of breath and movement.

By incorporating these chair yoga poses into your practice, you can experience the physical, mental, and emotional benefits of yoga in a gentle and accessible way. Remember to listen to your body, modify poses as needed, and practice with mindfulness and intention to maximize the benefits of your chair yoga practice.

BREATHING TECHNIQUES IN CHAIR YOGA

Breathing techniques, or pranayama, play a vital role in chair yoga practice, helping to deepen relaxation, increase mindfulness, and enhance the mind-body connection. In this chapter, we'll explore the importance of breathing in chair yoga, introduce key breathing techniques, and discuss how to incorporate them into your practice.

Introduction to Chair Yoga Breathing

Breathing is a fundamental aspect of yoga practice, serving as a bridge between the body and the mind. In chair yoga, breath awareness and control are used to cultivate mindfulness, reduce stress, and enhance the flow of energy throughout the body. By focusing on the breath, practitioners can regulate their nervous system, calm the mind, and deepen their connection to the present moment.

In chair yoga, breath awareness begins with simply observing the natural rhythm of the breath as it flows in and out of the body. This mindfulness of breath serves as a foundation for more advanced breathing techniques, allowing practitioners to explore different patterns of breathing and their effects on the body and mind.

Chair Yoga Pranayama Techniques

1. Deep Belly Breathing: Also known as diaphragmatic breathing, deep belly breathing involves inhaling deeply through the nose, allowing the breath to expand the abdomen fully, and exhaling completely through the nose or mouth. This technique promotes relaxation, reduces stress, and increases oxygenation of the blood.

2. Equal Breathing (Sama Vritti): Equal breathing involves inhaling and exhaling for an equal count, such as inhaling for a count of four and exhaling for a count of four. This technique helps to balance the nervous system, calm the mind, and improve concentration and focus.

3. Alternate Nostril Breathing (Nadi Shodhana): Alternate nostril breathing involves alternating the flow of breath between the left and right nostrils by using the fingers to block one nostril at a time. This technique helps to balance the flow of energy in the body, promote mental clarity, and reduce anxiety and stress.

4. Ujjayi Breath (Victorious Breath): Ujjayi breath involves slightly constricting the back of the throat to create a gentle ocean-like sound as you breathe in and out through the nose. This technique enhances focus, calms the mind, and generates internal heat, making it particularly beneficial for warming up the body during chair yoga practice.

5. *Three-Part Breath (Dirga Pranayama):* Three-part breath involves consciously directing the breath into three distinct areas of the torso: the lower belly, the ribcage, and the chest. This technique promotes deep relaxation, expands lung capacity, and increases oxygenation of the blood.

6. *Sitali Breath (Cooling Breath):* Sitali breath involves inhaling through a rolled tongue or pursed lips, creating a cooling sensation in the mouth and throat, and exhaling through the nose. This technique helps to reduce body heat, calm the mind, and soothe the nervous system, making it especially useful for cooling down after physical activity.

Incorporating these chair yoga pranayama techniques into your practice can help deepen your awareness of breath, promote relaxation, and enhance the overall benefits of your chair yoga practice. Experiment with different techniques to discover which ones resonate most with you and incorporate them into your daily routine for optimal health and well-being.

CHAIR YOGA ROUTINES

Chair yoga routines offer a structured sequence of poses and breathing exercises designed to address specific needs and goals, such as increasing flexibility, reducing stress, or building strength. In this chapter, we'll explore four chair yoga routines that you can incorporate into your daily practice to promote overall health and well-being.

Gentle Morning Chair Yoga Routine

Starting your day with a gentle chair yoga routine can help awaken your body, calm your mind, and set a positive tone for the day ahead. This routine focuses on gentle stretches and energizing breathwork to invigorate the body and prepare you for the day ahead.

1. Seated Mountain Pose: Sit tall on the edge of your chair, with your feet flat on the floor and hands resting on your thighs. Close your eyes and take several deep breaths, grounding yourself and setting an intention for your practice.

2. Seated Side Stretch: Inhale and reach your right arm overhead, stretching up and over to the left side. Hold for a few breaths, then switch sides and repeat on the other side.

3. Seated Forward Bend: Inhale to lengthen your spine, then exhale and hinge forward at your hips, folding your torso over your thighs. Hold for a few breaths, then slowly roll back up to an upright position.

4. Seated Twist: Inhale to lengthen your spine, then exhale and twist to the right, placing your left hand on the outside of your right thigh and your right hand on the back of the chair. Hold for a few breaths, then repeat on the other side.

5. Deep Belly Breathing: Sit tall and place one hand on your belly and the other on your chest. Inhale deeply through your nose, feeling your belly rise, then exhale completely through your mouth, feeling your belly fall. Repeat for several breaths, focusing on the sensation of the breath moving in and out of your body.

6. Seated Sun Salutation: Inhale and sweep your arms overhead, then exhale and bring your hands down to heart center. Repeat for several rounds, syncing your breath with your movement.

7. Closing Meditation: Close your practice with a few moments of seated meditation, focusing on your breath and allowing any tension or stress to melt away.

Chair Yoga for Stress Relief

Chair yoga can be a powerful tool for managing stress and promoting relaxation. This routine focuses on gentle stretches, calming breathwork, and mindfulness practices to help reduce stress and cultivate a sense of inner peace and tranquility.

1. *Equal Breathing:* Sit tall and inhale for a count of four, then exhale for a count of four. Repeat for several rounds, focusing on the rhythm of your breath and allowing your mind to become calm and steady.

2. *Seated Cat-Cow Stretch:* Inhale to arch your back and lift your chest (Cow Pose), then exhale to round your spine and tuck your chin to your chest (Cat Pose). Continue flowing between these two poses with your breath for several rounds.

3. *Seated Forward Bend with Breath Awareness:* Inhale to lengthen your spine, then exhale and fold forward at your hips, bringing your torso toward your thighs. Hold for a few breaths, then focus on sending your breath into any areas of tension or tightness in your body.

4. *Alternate Nostril Breathing:* Sit tall and use your right thumb to close your right nostril, then inhale deeply through your left nostril. Close your left nostril with your right ring finger, then exhale completely through your right nostril. Continue alternating between inhaling through the left nostril and exhaling through the right nostril for several rounds.

5. *Seated Twist with Mindfulness:* Inhale to lengthen your spine, then exhale and twist to the right, placing your left hand on the outside of your right thigh and your right hand on the back of the chair. As you hold the twist, bring your awareness to the sensation of your breath moving in and out of your body, and observe any thoughts or emotions that arise without judgment. Repeat on the other side.

6. Deep Belly Breathing: Close your practice with several rounds of deep belly breathing, focusing on the calming effect of the breath and allowing yourself to fully relax and let go of any tension or stress.

Chair Yoga for Flexibility

Flexibility is essential for maintaining mobility and preventing injury as we age. This chair yoga routine focuses on gentle stretches and range of motion exercises to improve flexibility and mobility in the muscles and joints.

1. Seated Shoulder Rolls: Sit tall and inhale as you lift your shoulders up toward your ears, then exhale and roll them back and down. Repeat for several rounds, moving with your breath and releasing any tension in your shoulders and neck.

2. Seated Side Stretch: Inhale to reach your right arm overhead, stretching up and over to the left side. Hold for a few breaths, then switch sides and repeat on the other side.

3. Seated Hamstring Stretch: Extend your right leg out in front of you, heel on the floor and toes pointing up. Inhale to lengthen your spine, then exhale and hinge forward at your hips, reaching toward your toes. Hold for a few breaths, then switch sides and repeat on the other side.

4. Seated Spinal Twist: Inhale to lengthen your spine, then exhale and twist to the right, placing your left hand on the outside of your right thigh and your right hand on the back of the chair. Hold for a few breaths, then repeat on the other side.

5. *Seated Hip Opener*: Cross your right ankle over your left knee, flexing your right foot to protect your knee. Inhale to lengthen your spine, then exhale and gently press down on your right knee to open up your hip. Hold for a few breaths, then switch sides and repeat on the other side.

6. *Seated Forward Bend*: Inhale to lengthen your spine, then exhale and hinge forward at your hips, bringing your chest toward your thighs. Hold for a few breaths, then slowly roll back up to an upright position.

7. *Deep Belly Breathing:* Close your practice with several rounds of deep belly breathing, allowing your breath to deepen and your body to relax into the stretches.

Chair Yoga for Strength

Building strength is essential for maintaining independence and vitality as we age. This chair yoga routine focuses on strengthening the muscles of the core, legs, and arms to improve stability, balance, and overall functional fitness.

1. Seated Leg Lifts: Sit tall and hold onto the sides of the chair for support. Inhale to lift your right leg straight out in front of you, engaging your core and quadriceps. Hold for a few breaths, then exhale to lower your leg back down. Repeat on the other side.

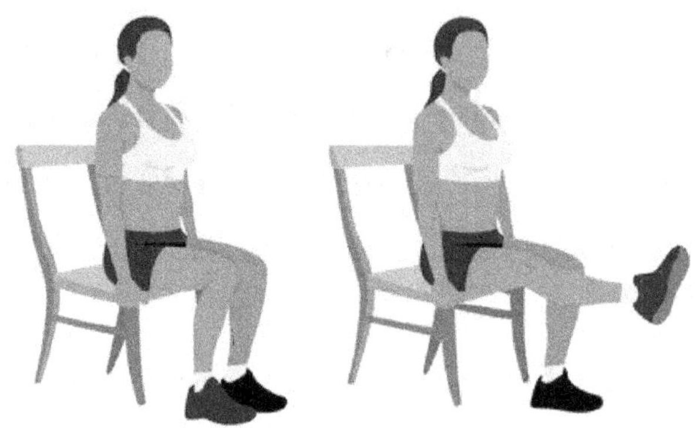

2. Seated Knee Raises: Sit tall and hold onto the sides of the chair for support. Inhale to lift your right knee toward your chest, engaging your core and hip flexors. Hold for a few breaths, then exhale to lower your knee back down. Repeat on the other side.

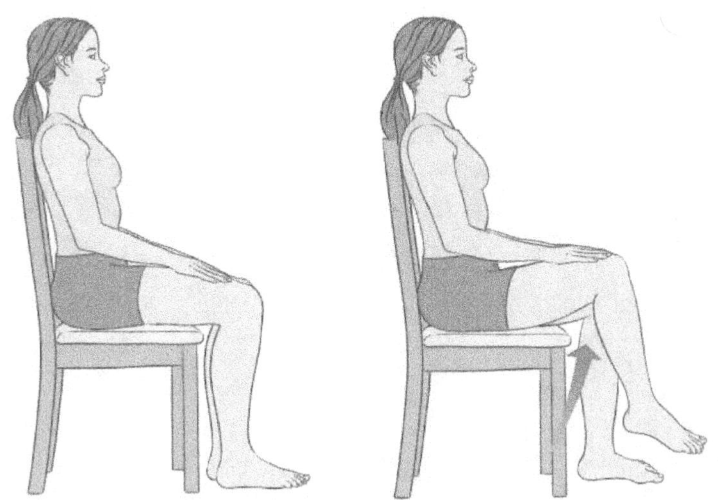

3. Seated Row: Sit tall and hold onto the sides of the chair for support. Inhale as you squeeze your shoulder blades together and pull your elbows back, bringing your hands toward your chest. Exhale to release and extend your arms forward. Repeat for several rounds, focusing on engaging the muscles of the upper back and arms.

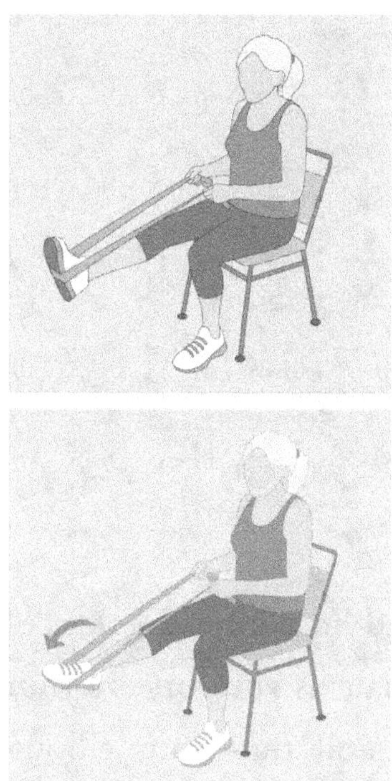

4. *Seated Chair Pose*: Sit tall on the edge of your chair with your feet flat on the floor and knees bent at a 90-degree angle. Inhale to lengthen your spine, then exhale and engage your core as you lift your hips a few inches off the chair, coming into a seated version of Chair Pose. Hold for a few breaths, then exhale to lower back down. Repeat for several rounds, focusing on building strength in the legs and core.

5. *Seated Bicep Curls*: Sit tall and hold onto a pair of light dumbbells or water bottles in each hand. Inhale as you bend your elbows and curl the weights toward your shoulders, engaging your biceps. Exhale to lower the weights back down. Repeat for several rounds, focusing on controlled movement and engaging the muscles of the arms.

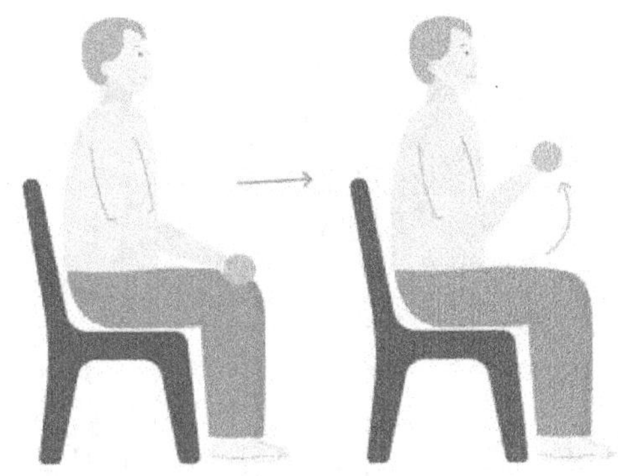

6. Seated Tricep Dips: Sit tall on the edge of your chair with your hands gripping the sides of the seat. Inhale to lift your hips off the chair, then exhale to bend your elbows and lower your hips toward the floor. Inhale to straighten your arms and lift your hips back up. Repeat for several rounds, focusing on engaging the muscles of the triceps and core.

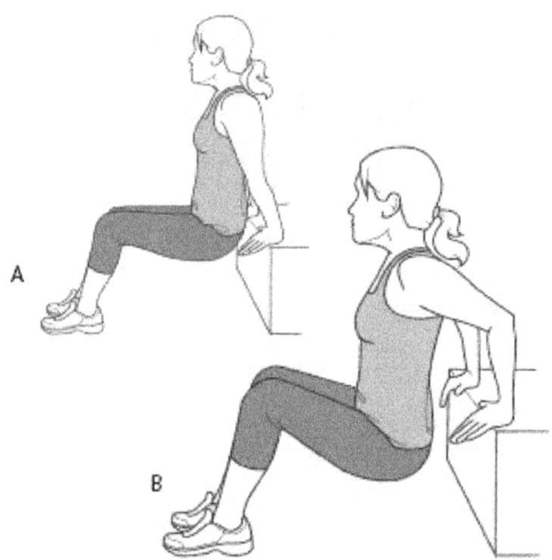

7. Seated Side Leg Lifts: Sit tall and hold onto the sides of the chair for support. Inhale to lift your right leg out to the side, engaging your outer thigh and hip abductors. Exhale to lower your leg back down. Repeat on the other side. Repeat for several rounds, focusing on engaging the muscles of the legs and hips.

8. Deep Belly Breathing: Close your practice with several rounds of deep belly breathing, allowing your breath to deepen and your body to relax after the strength-building exercises.

Chair Yoga for Back Pain

Chair yoga can be highly beneficial for individuals suffering from back pain, offering gentle stretches and strengthening exercises that promote flexibility and alleviate discomfort. Here's how chair yoga can help with back pain:

1. Gentle Stretches: Chair yoga includes a variety of gentle stretches specifically targeting the back muscles, such as seated twists, forward bends, and side stretches. These movements help improve flexibility and release tension in the spine.

2. *Strengthening:* Certain chair yoga poses strengthen the muscles supporting the spine, including the core muscles, which play a crucial role in maintaining spinal stability. Strengthening these muscles can help alleviate back pain and prevent future episodes.

3. *Mindful Movement*: Mindful movement practices incorporated into chair yoga help individuals become more aware of their body alignment and movement patterns. This awareness can lead to improved posture, reduced strain on the back, and decreased likelihood of exacerbating existing back pain.

4. *Low-Impact Exercise:* Chair yoga is low-impact and can be adapted to suit individuals of all fitness levels and mobility restrictions. This makes it a safe and accessible option for those with back pain who may find traditional exercise challenging or uncomfortable.

Chair Yoga for Better Sleep

Chair yoga offers gentle and accessible practices that can help promote better sleep by reducing stress, calming the mind, and relaxing the body. Here's how chair yoga contributes to better sleep.

1. ***Relaxation Techniques***: Chair yoga incorporates relaxation techniques such as deep breathing, which can activate the body's relaxation response, easing tension and promoting a sense of calm conducive to sleep.

2. ***Stress Reduction:*** Practicing chair yoga before bedtime helps alleviate stress accumulated throughout the day, allowing the body and mind to unwind and prepare for restorative sleep.

3. ***Improved Circulation***: Gentle movements and stretches in chair yoga enhance blood circulation, promoting relaxation and

aiding in the release of tension, which can contribute to better sleep quality.

4. *Mindfulness Practices:* Chair yoga often incorporates mindfulness techniques, such as mindful breathing and body awareness, which can help quiet racing thoughts and induce a state of relaxation conducive to falling asleep.

5. *Muscle Relaxation***:** Chair yoga poses target areas prone to tension buildup, such as the neck, shoulders, and back, promoting muscle relaxation and alleviating discomfort that may interfere with sleep.

Chair Yoga for Energy and Vitality

Chair yoga offers an accessible way to boost energy and vitality, making it suitable for individuals of all ages and fitness levels. Here's how chair yoga can enhance energy and vitality:

1. *Dynamic Movements:* Chair yoga incorporates dynamic movements that stimulate circulation and activate the body, leading to increased energy levels.

2. *Breath Awareness*: Pranayama techniques practiced in chair yoga help regulate breath and oxygen flow, revitalizing the body and mind.

3. *Mindfulness:* Chair yoga encourages mindfulness and present-moment awareness, reducing stress and fatigue while promoting a sense of vitality.

4. *Strength Building*: Engaging in chair yoga poses that target core muscles and improve strength can boost overall energy levels and stamina.

5. *Flexibility:* Gentle stretches and movements in chair yoga release tension from the body, enhancing flexibility and promoting a sense of lightness and vitality.

Chair Yoga for Better Posture

Chair yoga offers various poses that can help improve posture by strengthening core muscles, increasing flexibility, and promoting body awareness. Here's how chair yoga can contribute to better posture:

1. Seated Mountain Pose: Engage abdominal muscles and lengthen the spine while sitting tall on the chair, promoting proper alignment and spinal health.

2. Chest-Opening Poses: Poses like Supta Baddha Konasana and Viparita Dandasana focus on opening the chest and stretching the shoulders, counteracting rounded shoulders and encouraging an upright posture.

3. Core Strengthening: Chair yoga poses that engage the core muscles, such as seated twists and leg lifts, help stabilize the spine and support proper posture.

4. *Spinal Alignment:* Gentle spinal twists and side stretches in chair yoga maintain flexibility and alignment, reducing strain on the spine and promoting a balanced posture.

5. *Mindful Awareness:* Chair yoga encourages mindfulness of body alignment and sensations, helping individuals become more aware of their posture throughout the day and making adjustments as needed.

Chair Yoga for Mindfulness and Meditation

Chair yoga provides an accessible way to practice mindfulness and meditation, even for those with limited mobility. Here's how chair yoga can be beneficial for cultivating mindfulness and incorporating meditation:

1. *Mindful Movement:* Chair yoga involves gentle movements coordinated with breath awareness, fostering mindfulness by encouraging practitioners to stay present in the moment.

2. *Breathing Techniques*: Incorporating pranayama (breathing exercises) during chair yoga sessions promotes relaxation and enhances mindfulness. Techniques like deep breathing and full arm circles with breath awareness help calm the mind and deepen the meditative experience.

3. *Guided Practices:* Many chair yoga classes and videos offer guided meditation sessions tailored to seated postures, making it easier for participants to focus on breath and sensations while remaining comfortable in their chairs.

4. *Body Scan:* Seated body scan meditations, where practitioners systematically bring attention to different parts of the body while seated, can be effectively integrated into chair yoga routines, promoting relaxation and mindfulness.

5. *Mindful Awareness:* Chair yoga encourages mindful awareness of body sensations, thoughts, and emotions, providing a gentle yet effective way to develop mindfulness skills that can be applied off the mat.

Chair Yoga Poses for Balance

Chair yoga offers various poses tailored to improve balance, making it suitable for individuals of all skill levels and physical abilities. Here are some chair yoga poses specifically designed to enhance balance:

1. *Seated Mountain Pose:* Sit with feet flat on the floor, spine tall, and hands resting on thighs. This pose encourages grounding and stability.

2. *Seated Forward Bend:* Sit forward on the chair with feet hip-width apart. Inhale, lengthen the spine, then exhale, hinge at the hips, and fold forward, allowing the torso to rest on or between the thighs. Hold for a few breaths to improve balance and flexibility.

3. *Seated Side Bend:* Sit on the edge of the chair with feet grounded. Inhale, lift arms overhead, and exhale, side bend to the right, placing the right hand on the chair's edge while reaching the left arm overhead. Repeat on the other side to promote balance on both sides of the body.

4. *Heel Raises:* Sit tall with feet flat on the floor. Inhale, lift heels off the ground, and exhale, lower them down. Repeat several times to strengthen ankles and improve proprioception.

5. *Mountain Pose Variation with Leg Lift:* Sit tall with feet flat on the floor. Inhale, lift one leg, extending it forward while keeping the foot flexed. Hold for a few breaths, then switch sides. This pose challenges balance and strengthens leg muscles.

By incorporating these chair yoga routines into your regular practice, you can improve your flexibility, reduce stress, build strength, and enhance your overall health and well-being. Remember to listen to your body, modify poses as needed, and practice with mindfulness and intention to maximize the benefits of your chair yoga practice.

MODIFYING CHAIR YOGA POSES

Chair yoga offers a versatile and adaptable approach to yoga practice, making it accessible to individuals of all ages, abilities, and fitness levels. In this chapter, we'll explore how to modify chair yoga poses to accommodate different abilities and needs, as well as how to use props to enhance and support your practice.

Adapting Poses for Different Abilities

One of the key benefits of chair yoga is its ability to be modified and adapted to suit a wide range of abilities and physical conditions. Whether you're recovering from an injury, managing a chronic condition, or simply new to exercise, there are ways to make chair yoga poses accessible and enjoyable for everyone. Here are some strategies for adapting poses for different abilities:

1. Adjusting Range of Motion: If you have limited flexibility or range of motion, you can modify poses by reducing the range of motion or intensity of the movement. For example, instead of reaching your arms overhead in Seated Mountain Pose, you can keep your hands on your thighs or at heart center.

2. Using Support: Chairs can provide valuable support and stability during chair yoga practice. You can use the backrest, seat, or arms of the chair for support during poses such as Seated Forward Bend or Seated Twist. Holding onto the chair for balance can also help during standing poses or balance exercises.

3. Adding Props: Props such as yoga blocks, straps, or pillows can be used to modify poses and make them more accessible. For example, you can place a block under your feet in Seated Forward

Bend to reduce strain on the hamstrings, or use a strap to extend your reach in Seated Twist.

4. *Seated vs. Standing Options:* Many chair yoga poses can be adapted for both seated and standing practice, allowing you to choose the option that best suits your needs and abilities. If standing poses are challenging, you can modify them by performing a seated version instead.

5. *Breath Awareness:* Regardless of your physical ability, everyone can benefit from practicing breath awareness and mindfulness in chair yoga. Focusing on the breath can help calm the mind, reduce stress, and enhance the mind-body connection, regardless of the specific poses you're practicing.

By adapting poses to suit your individual needs and abilities, you can enjoy the benefits of chair yoga practice while honoring your body and avoiding injury.

Using Props in Chair Yoga

Props are valuable tools in chair yoga practice, helping to support the body, deepen stretches, and enhance alignment. Here are some common props used in chair yoga and how they can be used to support your practice:

1. *Yoga Blocks:* Yoga blocks can be used to modify poses and provide support and stability. For example, you can place a block under your feet in Seated Forward Bend to reduce strain on the hamstrings, or use a block between your thighs in Seated Mountain Pose to engage the inner thighs and pelvic floor muscles.

2. *Yoga Straps:* Yoga straps are useful for extending your reach and deepening stretches. You can use a strap to reach for your feet in Seated

Forward Bend, or to bind your hands in Seated Twist for a deeper stretch.

3. Blankets or Pillows: Blankets or pillows can provide cushioning and support during seated poses or relaxation exercises. You can place a blanket under your hips for added support in seated poses, or use a pillow to support your head and neck during Savasana (relaxation pose).

4. Chair: The chair itself is a valuable prop in chair yoga practice, providing support and stability during standing poses, balance exercises, and seated poses. You can use the backrest, seat, or arms of the chair for support and stability as needed.

5. Bolster: Bolsters are long, cylindrical cushions that can be used to support the body in reclined or seated poses. You can use a bolster under your knees in Savasana to relieve pressure on the lower back, or place it behind your back for support in seated poses.

By incorporating props into your chair yoga practice, you can customize your practice to suit your individual needs and preferences, making it more comfortable, enjoyable, and effective.

In summary, modifying chair yoga poses and using props can make yoga practice accessible to individuals of all abilities and fitness levels. Whether you're recovering from an injury, managing a chronic condition, or simply new to exercise, chair yoga offers a gentle and adaptable approach to yoga practice that can be tailored to suit your unique needs and abilities. By honoring your body and practicing with mindfulness and intention, you can experience the many benefits of chair yoga practice, including improved flexibility, strength, balance, and relaxation.

INCORPORATING MINDFULNESS INTO CHAIR YOGA

Mindfulness is a key component of yoga practice, encouraging present-moment awareness, deepening the mind-body connection, and fostering a sense of inner peace and tranquility. In this chapter, we'll explore how to incorporate mindfulness into chair yoga, including mindful movement and chair yoga practices for stress reduction and relaxation.

Mindful Movement In Chair Yoga

Mindful movement involves bringing awareness and intention to each movement, breath, and sensation during yoga practice. In chair yoga, mindful movement can help you cultivate a deeper connection to your body, increase proprioception, and enhance the overall benefits of your practice. Here are some tips for incorporating mindful movement into your chair yoga practice:

1. Focus on the Breath: Begin each chair yoga practice by bringing your attention to your breath. Notice the sensation of the breath moving in and out of your body, and use the breath as a guide for your movements.

2. Move with Awareness: As you move through each pose, pay attention to the sensations in your body and any areas of tension or tightness. Move slowly and mindfully, allowing your breath to guide your movements and deepen your awareness.

3. Listen to Your Body: Honor your body's limits and avoid pushing yourself into discomfort or pain. If a pose doesn't feel right for you, feel free to modify or skip it altogether. Trust your body's wisdom and adjust your practice accordingly.

4. Stay Present: Keep your focus on the present moment, letting go of distractions and thoughts about the past or future. By staying present with your breath and body, you can deepen your mindfulness practice and experience greater peace and clarity.

5. Cultivate Gratitude: Throughout your practice, cultivate an attitude of gratitude for your body and the opportunity to practice yoga. Take moments to appreciate the sensations of movement, the rhythm of your breath, and the sense of connection to yourself and the world around you.

By incorporating mindful movement into your chair yoga practice, you can deepen your connection to your body, quiet the mind, and experience greater presence and peace in each moment.

Chair Yoga for Stress Reduction and Relaxation

Chair yoga offers numerous techniques for reducing stress and promoting relaxation, making it an ideal practice for managing the demands of everyday life. By incorporating gentle stretches, breathing exercises, and mindfulness practices, you can create a calming and rejuvenating chair yoga routine to help you unwind and de-stress. Here's a sample chair yoga sequence for stress reduction and relaxation:

1. Deep Belly Breathing: Begin by sitting tall on the edge of your chair, with your feet flat on the floor and hands resting on your thighs. Close your eyes and take several deep breaths, focusing on expanding your belly with each inhale and contracting it with each exhale. Continue for several rounds, allowing your breath to deepen and your body to relax.

2. Seated Forward Bend: Inhale to lengthen your spine, then exhale and hinge forward at your hips, folding your torso over your thighs. Let your arms hang loose or rest them on your thighs, and allow your head to hang heavy. Hold for several breaths, feeling the stretch in your spine and hamstrings, and letting go of any tension or stress.

3. Seated Cat-Cow Stretch: Inhale to arch your back and lift your chest (Cow Pose), then exhale to round your spine and tuck your chin to your chest (Cat Pose). Continue flowing between these two poses with your breath, allowing the movement to be slow and gentle.

4. Alternate Nostril Breathing: Sit tall and bring your right hand to your face, using your thumb to close your right nostril and your ring finger to close your left nostril. Inhale deeply through your left nostril, then close it with your ring finger and exhale through your right nostril. Continue alternating between inhaling through the left nostril and exhaling through the right nostril for several rounds, focusing on the soothing rhythm of your breath.

5. Seated Twist: Inhale to lengthen your spine, then exhale and twist to the right, placing your left hand on the outside of your right thigh and your right hand on the back of the chair. Hold for several breaths, feeling the gentle twist in your spine and the release of tension in your back and shoulders. Repeat on the other side.

6. Savasana (Relaxation Pose): Finally, come to a comfortable seated position on your chair, with your feet flat on the floor and your hands resting on your thighs. Close your eyes and allow your body to relax completely, letting go of any remaining tension or stress. Stay here for several minutes, focusing on your breath and allowing yourself to be fully present in the moment.

By incorporating these chair yoga practices for stress reduction and relaxation into your daily routine, you can cultivate a greater sense of calm, balance, and well-being in your life. Remember to practice with mindfulness and intention, and to listen to your body's needs as you move through each pose and breath. With consistent practice, you can harness the power of chair yoga to manage stress, promote relaxation, and enhance your overall quality of life.

CHAIR YOGA FOR SPECIFIC NEEDS

Chair yoga is a versatile practice that can be adapted to meet the specific needs of individuals of all ages, lifestyles, and physical abilities. In this chapter, we'll explore how chair yoga can be tailored to address the unique needs of seniors, office workers, and individuals with limited mobility.

Chair Yoga for Seniors

Seniors can benefit greatly from practicing chair yoga, as it offers gentle stretches, strength-building exercises, and relaxation techniques that can help maintain mobility, improve balance, and enhance overall well-being. Chair yoga for seniors focuses on gentle movements and poses that are accessible and safe for aging bodies. Here are some key considerations when practicing chair yoga for seniors:

1. Joint Mobility: Seniors may experience stiffness or limited range of motion in their joints due to aging or arthritis. Chair yoga poses should be gentle and emphasize slow, controlled movements to help improve joint mobility and flexibility.

2. Balance and Stability: Falls are a common concern for seniors, so chair yoga poses should incorporate balance and stability exercises to help prevent falls and improve overall stability. Poses such as Seated Mountain Pose and Seated Warrior Pose can help strengthen the muscles of the legs and core, improving balance and stability.

3. Mindfulness and Relaxation: Seniors may also benefit from incorporating mindfulness and relaxation techniques into their chair yoga practice to reduce stress, promote relaxation, and enhance mental well-being. Breathing exercises, guided relaxation, and meditation can help seniors cultivate a sense of calm and inner peace.

4. **Social Connection:** Chair yoga classes can provide seniors with an opportunity to socialize and connect with others in a supportive and inclusive environment. Group classes can foster a sense of community and belonging, which is important for overall health and well-being.

By practicing chair yoga regularly, seniors can improve their physical health, enhance their mental well-being, and enjoy a greater sense of vitality and independence as they age.

Chair Yoga for Office Workers

Office workers often spend long hours sitting at a desk, which can lead to stiffness, tension, and discomfort in the body. Chair yoga offers a convenient and effective way for office workers to stretch, release tension, and rejuvenate their bodies throughout the workday. Here are some chair yoga poses and practices specifically designed for office workers:

1. Desk Stretches: Incorporate simple stretches and movements into your daily routine to counteract the effects of prolonged sitting. Shoulder rolls, neck stretches, and wrist circles can help relieve tension and improve circulation in the upper body.

2. Seated Twists: Seated twists can help relieve tension in the spine, improve digestion, and increase energy levels. To perform a seated twist, sit tall in your chair and gently twist your torso to one side, placing one hand on the back of the chair and the other hand on your thigh. Hold for several breaths, then repeat on the other side.

3. Breathing Breaks: Take short breaks throughout the workday to practice deep breathing exercises and mindfulness techniques. Close your eyes, place one hand on your belly and the other hand on your chest, and take several slow, deep breaths, focusing on the sensation of the breath moving in and out of your body.

4. Ergonomic Support: Use props such as cushions, pillows, or yoga blocks to support your body and improve posture while sitting at your desk. Place a cushion behind your lower back for lumbar support, or use a yoga block under your feet to elevate them and reduce pressure on the lower back and hips.

5. Mindful Movement: Incorporate short chair yoga sequences into your workday to stretch and energize your body. Simple sequences such as Seated Sun Salutations or Gentle Chair Yoga Flow can help increase circulation, improve flexibility, and boost mood and productivity.

By integrating chair yoga into their daily routine, office workers can reduce stress, increase energy levels, and improve overall physical and mental well-being, even amidst a busy work schedule.

Chair Yoga for People with Limited Mobility

Chair yoga is an accessible and inclusive practice that can be adapted to meet the needs of individuals with limited mobility, including those with disabilities, injuries, or chronic health conditions. Chair yoga offers gentle stretches, strengthening exercises, and relaxation techniques that can help improve mobility, reduce pain, and enhance quality of life. Here are some considerations when practicing chair yoga for people with limited mobility:

1. Range of Motion: Chair yoga poses should be modified to accommodate limited range of motion in the joints or muscles. Gentle movements and supported stretches can help improve flexibility and increase range of motion over time.

2. Stability and Support: Use props such as chairs, cushions, or bolsters to provide stability and support during chair yoga practice. Props can help individuals with limited mobility feel safe and secure while exploring different poses and movements.

3. Breath Awareness: Encourage individuals with limited mobility to focus on their breath and cultivate mindfulness during chair yoga practice. Deep breathing exercises can help reduce stress, promote relaxation, and increase awareness of the body and mind.

4. Adaptive Poses: Modify traditional yoga poses to make them more accessible for individuals with limited mobility. For example, Seated Mountain Pose can be modified by placing a cushion under the hips for support, or Seated Forward Bend can be performed with the hands resting on the thighs instead of reaching for the feet.

5. Gentle Movement: Emphasize gentle, slow movements and supported stretches to prevent strain or injury. Encourage individuals to move within their comfort zone and avoid pushing themselves into discomfort or pain.

Chair Yoga for Weight Loss

By practicing chair yoga regularly, individuals with limited mobility can experience improvements in flexibility, strength, and overall well-being, while honoring their body's unique needs and limitations.

In conclusion, chair yoga offers a versatile and adaptable approach to yoga practice that can be tailored to meet the specific needs of seniors, office workers, and individuals with limited mobility. Whether you're looking to improve mobility, reduce stress, or simply enhance your overall well-being, chair yoga offers a gentle and accessible way to experience the many benefits of yoga practice, regardless of age, lifestyle, or physical ability.

CHAIR YOGA FOR DAILY LIFE

Chair yoga offers a convenient and accessible way to incorporate yoga into your daily routine, providing numerous benefits for physical health, mental well-being, and overall quality of life. In this chapter, we'll explore how you can integrate chair yoga into your daily life and maintain consistency and progression in your practice.

Integrating Chair Yoga into Your Routine

Chair yoga can be practiced virtually anywhere, making it easy to incorporate into your daily life, whether at home, at work, or while traveling. Here are some tips for integrating chair yoga into your routine:

1. Set Aside Time: Schedule regular times throughout the day to practice chair yoga, such as in the morning before starting your day, during breaks at work, or in the evening before bedtime. Consistency is key to establishing a regular practice and experiencing the full benefits of chair yoga.

2. Create a Dedicated Space: Designate a quiet, comfortable space in your home or workplace where you can practice chair yoga without distractions. Set up a chair, cushion, or yoga mat to support your practice, and add any props or accessories that enhance your comfort and enjoyment.

3. Start Small: If you're new to chair yoga or have limited time available, start with shorter practice sessions and gradually increase the duration and intensity of your practice over time. Even just a few minutes of chair yoga each day can make a significant difference in your physical and mental well-being.

4. Be Flexible: Be willing to adapt your chair yoga practice to fit your schedule and circumstances. If you're short on time, try incorporating mini-practices throughout the day, such as stretching at your desk or practicing deep breathing while waiting in line. Remember that every little bit counts towards your overall well-being.

5. Combine with Other Activities: Look for opportunities to integrate chair yoga into other activities or routines throughout your day. For example, you can practice deep breathing while commuting to work, perform seated stretches while watching TV, or incorporate mindfulness exercises into your daily chores.

6. Stay Mindful: Approach your chair yoga practice with mindfulness and intention, focusing on the present moment and fully engaging with each movement, breath, and sensation. Cultivate awareness of your body and mind, and practice with kindness and compassion towards yourself.

Tips for Consistency and Progression

Consistency is key to making progress in your chair yoga practice and experiencing long-term benefits. Here are some tips for staying consistent and progressing in your practice:

1. Set Realistic Goals: Establish achievable goals for your chair yoga practice, such as practicing for a certain number of days per week or increasing the duration of your practice over time. Break larger goals down into smaller, manageable steps to help maintain motivation and momentum.

2. Track Your Progress: Keep track of your chair yoga practice in a journal or calendar to monitor your progress and celebrate your achievements.

Note any changes or improvements you observe in your physical health, mental well-being, or overall quality of life as a result of your practice.

3. Find Accountability: Share your chair yoga goals with a friend, family member, or yoga buddy who can offer support, encouragement, and accountability. Consider joining a chair yoga class or online community where you can connect with others who share similar interests and goals.

4. Stay Flexible: Be flexible and adaptable in your approach to chair yoga practice, especially when faced with challenges or setbacks. If you miss a practice session or encounter obstacles, don't be too hard on yourself. Instead, acknowledge your efforts and commit to getting back on track as soon as possible.

5. Celebrate Progress: Celebrate your progress and accomplishments along the way, no matter how small or seemingly insignificant. Recognize the effort and dedication you put into your chair yoga practice, and take pride in the positive changes you experience in your body, mind, and spirit.

6. Seek Support: Don't hesitate to seek support and guidance from a qualified yoga instructor or healthcare professional if you have questions or concerns about your chair yoga practice. A knowledgeable teacher can offer personalized guidance, modifications, and encouragement to help you reach your goals safely and effectively.

By integrating chair yoga into your daily routine and maintaining consistency and progression in your practice, you can experience the many benefits of yoga in your daily life, including improved flexibility, strength, balance, and overall well-being. Remember to approach your practice with an open mind and a compassionate heart, and to enjoy the journey of self-discovery and self-care that chair yoga offers.

FREQUENTLY ASKED QUESTIONS ABOUT CHAIR YOGA

Chair yoga is a gentle and accessible form of yoga that can benefit individuals of all ages and abilities. However, like any new practice, it's common to have questions and concerns when starting out. In this chapter, we'll address some frequently asked questions about chair yoga, common concerns, misconceptions, and how to troubleshoot common issues.

Common Concerns and Misconceptions

Q. Is chair yoga suitable for everyone?

A. Chair yoga is generally safe and accessible for people of all ages and fitness levels, including seniors, office workers, and individuals with limited mobility or injuries. However, it's important to listen to your body and modify poses as needed to suit your individual needs and abilities.

Q. *Will chair yoga provide the same benefits as traditional yoga?*

A. While chair yoga may not offer the same level of intensity or challenge as traditional yoga, it still provides numerous benefits for physical health, mental well-being, and overall quality of life. Chair yoga can improve flexibility, strength, balance, and relaxation, making it an effective practice for maintaining health and vitality.

Q. *Do I need to be flexible to practice chair yoga?*

A. No, you don't need to be flexible to practice chair yoga. Chair yoga poses can be modified to accommodate any level of flexibility or range of motion, making it accessible to people of all abilities. The focus is on gentle movements, breath awareness, and mindfulness, rather than achieving advanced yoga poses.

Q. Can I practice chair yoga if I have a health condition or injury?

A. In most cases, chair yoga can be practiced safely with a wide range of health conditions or injuries. However, it's important to consult with a healthcare professional before starting any new exercise program, especially if you have specific health concerns or medical conditions. Your healthcare provider can offer personalized guidance and recommendations based on your individual needs.

Troubleshooting Common Issues

1. Difficulty with balance or stability: If you're having trouble with balance or stability during chair yoga practice, try using props such as a wall, chair, or yoga blocks for support. Focus on engaging your core muscles and maintaining a steady breath to improve stability.

2. Feeling discomfort or strain in certain poses: If you're experiencing discomfort or strain in certain poses, try modifying the pose to make it more accessible or comfortable for your body. Use props such as cushions or pillows for support, and avoid pushing yourself into pain or discomfort. Listen to your body and honor its limits.

3. Difficulty focusing or staying present during practice: If you're having trouble staying focused or present during chair yoga practice, try incorporating mindfulness techniques such as deep breathing, body scanning, or guided visualization. Bring your attention back to your breath whenever your mind starts to wander, and practice with a sense of curiosity and openness.

4. Lack of motivation or consistency in practice: If you're struggling to stay motivated or consistent in your chair yoga practice, try setting realistic goals, creating a dedicated space for practice, and finding accountability through a friend, family member, or yoga buddy. Remember to celebrate your progress and acknowledge the positive impact of your practice on your physical and mental well-being.

5. Feeling self-conscious or insecure about practicing chair yoga: If you're feeling self-conscious or insecure about practicing chair yoga, remember that yoga is a personal journey and there's no judgment or competition in yoga practice. Focus on your own experience and listen to your body's needs without comparing yourself to others. Embrace your unique journey and trust in the transformative power of chair yoga to support your health and well-being.

By addressing common concerns, misconceptions, and troubleshooting common issues, you can feel more confident and empowered to embark on your chair yoga journey with clarity, ease, and joy. Remember to approach your practice with an open mind, a compassionate heart, and a sense of curiosity and exploration, and to enjoy the many benefits that chair yoga has to offer for your body, mind, and spirit.

CONCLUSION

As we come to the end of this journey through the world of chair yoga, it's important to reflect on the key points we've covered and to offer encouragement for continuing your chair yoga practice.

Recap of Key Points

Throughout this book, we've explored the many benefits of chair yoga, including improved flexibility, strength, balance, and relaxation. We've learned how chair yoga can be adapted to meet the needs of individuals of all ages, abilities, and lifestyles, making it accessible and inclusive for everyone. We've discussed how to integrate chair yoga into your daily routine, troubleshoot common issues, and address concerns and misconceptions about the practice.

Some of the key points we've covered include:

1. **Accessibility**: Chair yoga is accessible to people of all ages and abilities, including seniors, office workers, and individuals with limited mobility or injuries.

2. **Adaptability**: Chair yoga poses can be modified to accommodate any level of flexibility or range of motion, making it suitable for beginners and experienced practitioners alike.

3. **Benefits**: Chair yoga offers numerous benefits for physical health, mental well-being, and overall quality of life, including improved flexibility, strength, balance, and relaxation.

4. **Mindfulness**: Chair yoga emphasizes mindfulness and breath awareness, helping to cultivate present-moment awareness, reduce stress, and enhance the mind-body connection.

5. **Consistency**: Consistency is key to experiencing the full benefits of chair yoga. By integrating chair yoga into your daily routine and practicing regularly, you can maintain physical health, mental well-being, and overall vitality.

Encouragement for Continuing Your Chair Yoga Practice

As you continue your chair yoga practice, I encourage you to approach it with an open mind, a compassionate heart, and a sense of curiosity and exploration. Remember that yoga is a personal journey, and there's no right or wrong way to practice. Listen to your body, honor its limits, and practice with kindness and self-compassion.

Be patient with yourself and celebrate your progress along the way, no matter how small or seemingly insignificant. Every moment spent on your mat is an opportunity for growth, learning, and self-discovery. Embrace the challenges and the victories, and trust in the transformative power of chair yoga to support your health and well-being.

Seek support and guidance from qualified teachers, mentors, and fellow practitioners as needed, and remember that you're never alone on your yoga journey. Share your experiences, insights, and challenges with others, and be open to learning from their wisdom and perspectives.

Above all, continue to nourish your body, mind, and spirit through the practice of chair yoga. Cultivate gratitude for the opportunity to practice, and let your practice be a source of joy, inspiration, and empowerment in your life.

Thank you for joining me on this journey through the world of chair yoga. May your practice be filled with peace, vitality, and abundant blessings, now and always. *Namaste.*

ADDITIONAL RESOURCES

In this final chapter, we'll explore additional resources that can support your journey with chair yoga, including books, websites, apps, and how to find chair yoga classes near you.

Books for Further Learning

1. *"Chair Yoga: Sit, Stretch, and Strengthen Your Way to a Happier, Healthier You"* by Kristin McGee: This comprehensive guide offers a variety of chair yoga poses and sequences suitable for all levels, along with tips for incorporating mindfulness and relaxation techniques into your practice.

2. *"Every Body Yoga: Let Go of Fear, Get On the Mat, Love Your Body"* by Jessamyn Stanley: While not specifically focused on chair yoga, this empowering book offers valuable insights and

inspiration for anyone interested in yoga, regardless of body shape, size, or ability.

3. *"Yoga for Healthy Aging: A Guide to Lifelong Well-Being"* by Baxter Bell and Nina Zolotow: This informative book provides valuable guidance on adapting yoga practices for older adults, including chair yoga sequences and modifications for various health conditions.

Websites and Apps

1. **Yoga International** (https://www.yogainternational.com): This website offers a wide range of online yoga classes, including chair yoga classes suitable for all levels. You can choose from a variety of styles and instructors to find the perfect class for your needs.

2.   **Down**   **Dog**   **App** (https://www.downdogapp.com): This popular yoga app offers customizable yoga classes that you can tailor to your preferences, including chair yoga options. With options to adjust difficulty, duration, and focus area, you can create the perfect chair yoga practice for your needs.

3. **YouTube**: There are numerous YouTube channels dedicated to chair yoga, offering free videos ranging from gentle stretches to full-length classes. Some popular channels include Yoga With Adriene, SarahBethYoga, and Chair Yoga with Sherry Zak Morris.

Finding Chair Yoga Classes Near You

1. **Local Yoga Studios:** Many yoga studios offer chair yoga classes as part of their regular class schedule. Check with studios in your area to see if

they offer chair yoga classes and inquire about class times, instructors, and pricing.

2. **Senior Centers:** Senior centers often offer chair yoga classes tailored specifically for older adults. These classes may be offered on a drop-in basis or as part of a structured program. Contact your local senior center for more information.

3. **Community Centers:** Community centers, recreation centers, and libraries may also offer chair yoga classes as part of their wellness programming. Check their class schedules or websites for information on upcoming classes and registration.

4. **Online Directories:** Use online directories such as YogaFinder (https://www.yogafinder.com) or Mindbody (https://www.mindbodyonline.com) to search for chair yoga classes in your area. You can filter

results by location, class type, and instructor to find classes that meet your preferences.

5. Word of Mouth: Ask friends, family members, or healthcare providers for recommendations on chair yoga classes in your area. Personal recommendations can be a valuable resource for finding high-quality classes that meet your needs and preferences.

By exploring these additional resources, you can deepen your understanding of chair yoga, access a variety of practices and teachings, and find classes that support your journey to health and well-being. Whether you prefer learning through books, websites, apps, or in-person classes, there are resources available to help you on your path with chair yoga.

www.ingramcontent.com/pod-product-compliance
Lightning Source LLC
Chambersburg PA
CBHW081218260726
48653CB00010BB/3682